HOLT

Decisions for Health

LEVEL RED

Decision-Making and Refusal Skills Workbook

HOLT, RINEHART AND WINSTON
A Harcourt Education Company
Orlando • **Austin** • New York • San Diego • Toronto • London

TO THE STUDENT

This workbook contains Decision-Making and Refusal Skills worksheets for each chapter. These worksheets are designed to help you practice the life skills, "Making Good Decisions" and "Using Refusal Skills." By practicing these life skills with this workbook, you can prepare yourself to use these skills when faced with real-life decisions and circumstances.

Cover photo: G. Russ Images

Printed in the United States of America

ISBN 0-03-068351-3
1 2 3 4 5 6 7 170 07 06 05 04 03

Contents

A Healthy Body, a Healthy Weight

Decision-Making Skills Worksheets

Refusal Skills Worksheets

Mental and Emotional Health

Decision-Making Skills Worksheets

Refusal Skills Worksheets

Managing Stress

Decision-Making Skills Worksheets

Refusal Skills Worksheets

Encouraging Healthy Relationships

Decision-Making Skills Worksheets

Refusal Skills Worksheets

Conflict and Violence

Decision-Making Skills Worksheets

Refusal Skills Worksheets

Teens and Tobacco

Teens and Alcohol

Teens and Drugs

Infectious Diseases

Noninfectious Diseases and Disorders

Your Changing Body

Decision-Making Skills Worksheets

Refusal Skills Worksheets

Your Personal Safety

Decision-Making Skills Worksheets

Refusal Skills Worksheets

Name ________________________ Class ______________ Date ____________

Skills Worksheet

Decision-Making Skills

Lesson: Making Good Health Choices

Read the following scenario. Then, follow the steps below to decide what you would do in this situation.

It is a beautiful Saturday afternoon. Your homework is done, your chores are finished, and you have some free time. You are trying to decide which friend to call. If you call your friend Tim, he's sure to want to play soccer or ride bicycles. If you call your friend Matt, he'll probably want to watch television or play video games.

1. **Identify the problem.** What decision do you have to make?

   ____

   ____

2. **Consider your values.** What is important to you?

   ____

   ____

3. **List the options.** What possible actions could you take?

   ____

   ____

   ____

4. **Weigh the consequences.** List the pros and cons of each option.

   ____

   ____

   ____

5. **Decide and act.** Describe what you will do. Explain your decision.

   ____

   ____

6. **Evaluate your choice.** How do you feel about the action you took? Did you make a good decision? Would you take a different action if faced with the same scenario again?

   ____

   ____

Name ______________________ Class ______________ Date ____________

Skills Worksheet

Decision-Making Skills

Lesson: Nine Life Skills for Better Health

Pretend that you write an advice column for students that appears in the newspaper. Read the following letter. Then, write your response.

Dear Advice Guy,

I am a seventh-grader with a big problem. I always seem to be arguing with my younger sister, Clara. I want to get along better with her, but I'm not sure how. One friend suggested that I spend more time with her, but another friend told me that I should just ignore her. How can I decide what to do? And how will I know if the choice I make is working?

Clueless About Clara

Name ______________________ Class ____________ Date ____________

Skills Worksheet

Refusal Skills

Lesson: Influences on Your Health

Describe how you would use the following refusal skills to respond to the following scenario. Remember to be clear and choose your words carefully. Describe your body language as well as your words.

You have asthma. You know from past experience that just being around tobacco smoke can bring on an asthma attack. At a party, your friends, Becky and Ryan, want you to join them on the patio while they smoke cigarettes. You are worried that the smoke might bother you. However, you don't want Becky and Ryan to think that you're being unfriendly.

1. **Say no.** How would you say no to Becky and Ryan?

____

____

2. **Offer an alternative.** What else could you do with Becky and Ryan?

____

____

3. **Stand your ground.** What would you do if Becky and Ryan kept pressuring you to join them while they smoke?

____

____

4. **Walk away.** Describe how you would get out of the situation.

____

____

5. **Plan ahead.** What could you do to avoid this situation? Who can help you practice refusing this action?

____

____

6. **Have a support system.** Who will stand by you when you make this decision? How can you use these people as support when refusing to do this action?

____

____

Name ______________________________ Class ________________ Date ____________

Skills Worksheet

Refusal Skills

Lesson: Making Good Health Choices

Finish the story on the lines that follow. Explain how Mario could use refusal skills to respond to the scenario. Describe his actions as well as his words.

Mario never used to think about making good health choices. Last year, though, his sister was seriously hurt in a car accident because she wasn't wearing a seat belt. Since then, Mario has had a new attitude. He takes better care of himself, and he always buckles up when riding in the car. Yesterday, however, Mario's older cousin Jeff was supposed to give him a ride to the game. When Mario got in the car and started to buckle his seat belt, Jeff laughed and said, "What's up? You afraid to ride with me? Are you trying to insult my driving?" Then, Jeff told Mario to forget about using the seat belt.

Name ______________________ Class ______________ Date ______________

Skills Worksheet

Decision-Making Skills

Lesson: Six Steps to Making Good Decisions

Read the following situation. Then, follow the steps below to decide what you would do in this situation.

You promised to help your friend Shareen paint her bedroom on Saturday. She is excited about fixing up her room. She has been talking about it all week. On Friday, your friend Josh asks you to go with him to a movie on Saturday instead. The movie sounds like more fun, but you already made a commitment to Shareen.

1. **Identify the problem.** What decision do you have to make?

____

____

2. **Consider your values.** What is important to you?

____

____

3. **List the options.** What possible actions could you take?

____

____

4. **Weigh the consequences.** List the pros and cons of each option.

____

____

____

5. **Decide and act.** Describe what you will do. Explain your decision.

____

____

____

6. **Evaluate your choice.** How do you feel about the action you took? Did you make a good decision? Would you take a different action if faced with the same scenario again?

____

____

____

Name ______________________ Class ____________ Date ____________

Skills Worksheet

Decision-Making Skills

Lesson: Influences on Your Decisions

Pretend that you write an advice column for students that appears in the local newspaper. Read the following letter. Then, write your response in the space provided.

Dear Advice Guy,

I am a seventh-grader with a big problem. My parents gave me a gift certificate to my favorite clothing store for my birthday. My friend thinks I should use it to buy two or three T-shirts with the names of bands on front. However, we're not allowed to wear those kinds of T-shirts to school. I know my parents would rather I used the gift certificate for school clothes. I also really like some jeans I saw on a commercial last night, but they're expensive. I would only be able to afford one pair. What should I do?

Confused About Clothes

Name ______________________ Class ______________ Date ______________

Skills Worksheet

Refusal Skills

Lesson: How to Reach Your Goals

Describe how you would use refusal skills to respond to the following scenario. Remember to be clear and choose your words carefully. Describe your body language as well as your words.

Your goal is to make the school track team. To do that, you know that you will need to get faster and stronger, so you run after school every day. Two friends, Katie and Jason, constantly put down your efforts, though. They say your goal is unrealistic, and they make fun of you for working so hard. One afternoon, they walk up just as you are getting ready for your run. They say they are going to the park to hang out, and they ask you to join them.

1. **Say no.** How would you say no to Katie and Jason?

____

____

2. **Offer an alternative.** What else could you do with Katie and Jason?

____

____

3. **Stand your ground.** What would you do if they kept pressuring you to go to the park?

____

____

4. **Walk away.** Describe how you would get out of the situation.

____

____

5. **Plan ahead.** What could you do to avoid this situation? Who can help you practice refusing this action?

____

____

6. **Have a support system.** Who will stand by you when you make this decision? How can you use these people as support when refusing to do this action?

____

____

Name ________________________ Class ______________ Date ____________

Skills Worksheet

Refusal Skills

Lesson: Changing Your Goals

Finish the story on the lines that follow. Tell how Maria might want to change her goal. Also, explain how she could use refusal skills to respond to the scenario. Describe her body language as well as her words.

Maria's goal was to get the lead role in the class play. She learned her lines for the tryout, and she practiced every day after school for three weeks. On the day of the tryout, she did quite well. However, although she got a good part, it was not the starring role. Maria was crushed. Her friends, Jake and Christina, told her not to take the smaller part. They said it was a waste of her time. Instead, Jake and Christina said Maria should hang out with them at the mall after school.

Name ______________________ Class ______________ Date ____________

Skills Worksheet

Decision-Making Skills

Lesson: Self-Esteem and Your Life

Read the following situation. Then, follow the steps below to decide what you would do in this situation.

You are running for office on the student council. The race is close, and there are only two days left until students vote. You overhear a rumor about your opponent. You know if you spread the rumor, you will win the election.

1. **Identify the problem.** What decision do you have to make?

____

____

2. **Consider your values.** What is important to you?

____

____

3. **List the options.** What possible actions could you take?

____

____

4. **Weigh the consequences.** List the pros and cons of each option.

____

____

5. **Decide and act.** Describe what you will do. Explain your decision.

____

____

6. **Evaluate your choice.** How do you feel about the action you took? Did you make a good decision? Would you take a different action if faced with the same scenario again?

____

____

Name ______________________ Class ______________ Date ______________

Skills Worksheet

Decision-Making Skills

Lesson: Keys to Healthy Self-Esteem

Read the following situation. Then, follow the steps below to decide what you would do in this situation.

The big game between your school and your school's biggest rival just ended. Your team lost. As you and a group of your friends are leaving the school grounds, you notice the other team's bus. No one is near it. Your friends think that vandalizing the bus would be a good way to get back at the other team. You're not so sure that it's a good idea.

1. **Identify the problem.** What decision do you have to make?

____

____

2. **Consider your values.** What is important to you?

____

____

3. **List the options.** What possible actions could you take?

____

____

4. **Weigh the consequences.** List the pros and cons of each option.

____

____

5. **Decide and act.** Describe what you will do. Explain your decision.

____

____

6. **Evaluate your choice.** How do you feel about the action you took? Did you make a good decision? Would you take a different action if faced with the same scenario again?

____

____

Name ______________________ Class ______________ Date ______________

Skills Worksheet

Refusal Skills

Lesson: Your Self-Concept

Describe how you would use the following refusal skills to respond to the following scenario. Remember to be clear and choose your words carefully. Describe your body language as well as your words.

You and your new friend Leo are watching a video at Leo's house. Leo's parents are not home. A few minutes into the movie, Leo shows you a bag of marijuana. He says it's "really good stuff" and asks if you want to smoke some. When you say no, Leo starts to argue. He says things like "Come on. Who's gonna know?" "What's the big deal ?" and "Hey, if we get caught, I'll take all the blame."

1. **Say no.** How would you say no to Leo?

____

____

2. **Offer an alternative.** What else could you and Leo do?

____

____

3. **Stand your ground.** What would you do if Leo kept pressuring you to try marijuana?

____

____

4. **Walk away.** Describe how you would get out of the situation.

____

____

5. **Plan ahead.** What could you do to avoid this situation? Who can help you practice refusing marijuana and resisting peer pressure?

____

____

6. **Have a support system.** Who will stand by you when you make this decision? Who can you turn to for support when you refuse to smoke with Leo?

____

____

Name ______________________ Class ______________ Date ____________

Skills Worksheet

Refusal Skills

Lesson: Keys to Healthy Self-Esteem

Read the following situation, and write an ending using refusal skills.

Your book report is due in two days. You've read the book, and you've just started writing your report. Your friend Royce comes by and reminds you that you promised to go to the basketball tournament with her. The tournament will go on for the next two days, and your school is expected to win. When you tell Royce that you have to stay home and write your book report, she says, "Oh, no you don't. I'll give you a report that my sister wrote when she was in our class. I found it in an old notebook. You can just copy it. She got a B on it!"

Name ______________________ Class ______________ Date ____________

Skills Worksheet

Decision-Making Skills

Lesson: Your Fitness Program

Read the following situation. Then, follow the steps below to decide what you should do in this situation.

Imagine that your physical education teacher tested your fitness in September. You met healthy fitness zones for flexibility. However, you didn't meet the healthy fitness zones for pull-ups, curl-ups, and the 1-mile run. Your teacher is having another fitness test in March.

1. **Identify the problem.** What decision do you have to make?

   ____

2. **Consider your values.** What is important to you?

   ____

   ____

3. **List the options.** What possible actions could you take?

   ____

   ____

4. **Weigh the consequences.** List the pros and cons of each option.

   ____

   ____

   ____

5. **Decide and act.** Describe what you will do.Explain your decision.

   ____

   ____

   ____

6. **Evaluate your choice.** How do you feel about the action you took? Did you make a good decision? Would you take a different action if faced with the same scenario again?

   ____

   ____

   ____

Name ______________________ Class ______________ Date ____________

Skills Worksheet

Decision-Making Skills

Lesson: Eight Ways to Avoid Injury

Read the following situation. Then, follow the steps below to decide what you should do in this situation.

Imagine that you are on your school's track team. You need a new pair of running shoes. So, you and your parents go shopping. You narrow it down to two pairs of shoes. One pair seems a bit too small, but it is less expensive. The other pair is more comfortable, but it costs much more. Which pair should you get?

1. **Identify the problem.** What decision do you have to make?

____

2. **Consider your values.** What is important to you?

____

____

3. **List the options.** What possible actions could you take?

____

____

____

4. **Weigh the consequences.** List the pros and cons of each option.

____

____

5. **Decide and act.** Describe what you will do. Explain your decision.

____

____

____

6. **Evaluate your choice.** How do you feel about the action you took? Did you make a good decision? Would you take a different action if faced with the same scenario again?

____

____

Name ______________________ Class ______________ Date ____________

Skills Worksheet

Refusal Skills

Lesson: Sports and Competition

Read the journal entry below. Then, write a journal entry describing how you would use your refusal skills in this situation.

Saturday

Dear Journal,

I had a soccer game today. Some of my teammates were acting really badly. They booed at kids on the other team, played dirty, yelled at at the refs, and didn't shake hands after the game. I know this is the wrong way to act when you are playing sports. Doing all this doesn't really help you win the game. Now, some of my teammates want me to do the same thing.

Tuesday

Dear Journal,

____

____

____

____

____

____

____

____

____

____

____

____

____

____

____

____

Name ______________________ Class ______________ Date ____________

Skills Worksheet

Refusal Skills

Lesson: Eight Ways to Avoid Injury

Describe how Samantha could use refusal skills to respond to the following scenario. Remember to be clear and choose your words carefully. Describe her body language as well as her words.

Samantha runs for her school's track team. State finals are coming up soon, and her relay team really wants to go to the finals. To get ready, Samantha's teammates are working out more often and for longer periods of time even though her coach told them not to. Samantha knows that too much exercise can lead to injury. But her teammates want her to do the same workouts.

1. **Say no.** How could Samantha say no to her teammates?

____

____

2. **Offer an alternative.** What else could they do to improve their performance?

____

____

3. **Stand your ground.** What could Samantha do if her friends keep pressuring her?

____

____

4. **Walk away.** Describe how she could get out of the situation.

____

____

5. **Plan ahead.** What could Samantha do to avoid this situation? Who can help her practice refusing this action?

____

____

6. **Have a support system.** Who will stand by Samantha when she makes this decision? How could she use these people as support when refusing to do this action?

____

____

Name ______________________ Class ____________ Date ____________

Skills Worksheet

Decision-Making Skills

Lesson: Nutrition and Diet

Read the following situation. Then, follow the steps below to decide what you would do in this situation.

In between doing your homework and going to football practice, you decide to have a snack. The last slice of apple pie is on the kitchen counter and your favorite ice cream is in the freezer. You aren't really hungry but you want to munch on something to help boost your energy. You head to the kitchen to fix a snack, but you notice next to the pie is a bowl of fresh fruit.

1. **Identify the problem.** What decision do you have to make?

____

____

2. **Consider your values.** What is important to you?

____

____

3. **List the options.** What possible actions could you take?

____

____

4. **Weigh the consequences.** List the pros and cons of each option.

____

____

5. **Decide and act.** Describe what you will do. Explain your decision.

____

____

6. **Evaluate your choice.** How do you feel about the action you took? Did you make a good decision?

____

____

Name ______________________ Class ______________ Date ____________

Skills Worksheet

Decision-Making Skills

Lesson: Balancing Your Diet

You are responsible for planning the menu for your diversity club fund-raiser dinner. Foods from each culture should be represented, and you will need to use the Food Guide Pyramid. Practice decision-making skills to create a menu. Remember to: *identify the problem, consider your values, list the options, weigh the consequences, decide and act,* and *evaluate your choice*. Write about each step you take in the decision-making process. Later, share your menu with the class.

Name ______________________ Class ______________ Date ____________

Skills Worksheet

Refusal Skills

Lesson: Balancing Your Diet

Describe how you would use the following refusal skills to respond to the following scenario. Remember to be clear and choose your words carefully. Describe your body language as well as your words.

You are invited to your friend Gina's house for dinner. Gina's mom is a great cook but sometimes she cooks meals that are high in fat and sodium. Your family eats more of a well-balanced diet so you decide to eat a smaller portion. Gina's mom thinks you're just being polite and decides to pile a heap of food on your plate without asking you first.

1. **Say no.** How would you say no to Gina's mom without seeming rude?

____

____

2. **Offer an alternative.** What else could you say?

____

____

3. **Stand your ground.** What else might you do if Gina's mom insists?

____

____

4. **Walk away.** Describe how you would get out of the situation.

____

____

5. **Plan ahead.** What could you do to avoid this situation? Who can help you practice refusing this action?

____

____

6. **Have a support system.** Who will stand by you when you make this decision? How can you use these people as support?

____

____

Name ______________________ Class ______________ Date ____________

Skills Worksheet

Refusal Skills

Lesson: Building Healthful Eating Habits

Every day we encounter nutrition choices. At popular fast-food restaurants we are often asked to upgrade our orders. Describe how you would use refusal skills in the following scenario. Remember to be clear and choose your words carefully.

Order Taker: Welcome like to Charlie's Take Out! May I take your order?

You: Yes, I'd like the burger with fries meal.

Order Taker: Would you like to upgrade your meal?

1. **You: Say No**. How would you say no to the extras?

____

____

Order Taker: Would you like cheese or our secret sauce?

2. **You: Offer an Alternative.** What else could you order on your burger?

____

____

Order Taker: What about dessert? Would you like a brownie hot fudge sundae?

3. **You: Stand your ground.** What would you say to the order taker if you're feeling pressured?

____

____

4. **Plan Ahead.** How could you order differently to avoid this situation?

____

____

5. **Walk away.** Can you feel confident about the choices you've made? Explain your answer.

____

____

6. **Have a support system.** Who will stand by you when you make this decision? How can these people support you when you are refusing something?

____

____

Name ______________________ Class ____________ Date ____________

Skills Worksheet

Decision-Making Skills

Lesson: Building a Healthy Body Image

Read the following situation. Then, follow the steps below to decide what you would do in this situation.

One day, your best friend comes over to your house after school. While the two of you are working on your homework, she pulls a magazine from her school bag and says that, if you lost some weight, you could look just like the celebrity on the cover of the magazine. Looking closely, you see that this celebrity appears to have practically no body fat. You compare your body to the celebrity's body, think about your friend's comments, and start to feel badly about your body.

1. **Identify the problem.** What decision do you have to make?

____

____

2. **Consider your values.** What is important to you?

____

____

3. **List the options.** What possible actions could you take?

____

____

4. **Weigh the consequences.** List the pros and cons of each option.

____

____

5. **Decide and act.** Describe what you will do. Explain your decision.

____

____

6. **Evaluate your choice.** How do you feel about the action you took? Did you make a good decision? Would you take a different action if faced with the same scenario again?

____

____

Name ______________________ Class ______________ Date ____________

Skills Worksheet

Decision-Making Skills

Lesson: Managing Your Weight

Imagine that you are an advice columnist. Read each of the following letters. Then, write a brief response to each letter.

1. Dear Weight Wizard,

I am a fourteen-year old boy. I want to lose some weight, but I want to do it in a healthy way. What can I do?

Signed,

Looking to Lose

Dear Looking to Lose,

____

____

____

____

____

____

2. Dear Weight Wizard,

I am fifteen years old. My parents say that being physically active is important. I know that this is true, but I don't really like playing sports. What advice can you give a girl like me?

Signed,

Not An Athlete

Dear Not An Athlete,

____

____

____

____

____

____

Name ______________________ Class ______________ Date ____________

Skills Worksheet

Refusal Skills

Lesson: Eating Disorders

Describe how you would use the following refusal skills to respond to the following scenario. Remember to be clear and choose your words carefully. Describe your body language as well as your words.

Your best friend calls and tells you that he or she has discovered a great plan for getting a "perfect" body. As your friend describes this plan, which includes pills and special drinks, you realize that it's a fad diet. After your friend explains the diet, he or she invites you to participate, too.

1. **Say no.** How would you say no to your friend?

____

____

____

2. **Offer an alternative.** How else could you and your friend work toward healthy bodies?

____

____

3. **Stand your ground.** What would you do if he or she kept pressuring you to try the diet?

____

____

4. **Walk away.** Describe how you would get out of the situation.

____

____

5. **Plan ahead.** What could you do to avoid this situation? Who can help you practice refusing this action?

____

____

6. **Have a support system.** Who will stand by you when you make this decision? How can you use these people as support when refusing to do this action?

____

____

Name ______________________ Class ______________ Date ____________

Skills Worksheet

Refusal Skills

Lesson: Managing Your Weight

Write an ending to the following scenario. Remember to be clear and choose your words carefully. Describe your body language as well as your words.

You and your parents are at a high school graduation party for your cousin Renee. There is a refreshment table at the back of the reception hall with snacks, beverages, and a variety of desserts. You notice a fruit salad, a tray of raw vegetable slices, bowls of potato chips, and cookies. You also see several types of soda, small bottles of water, and pitchers of fruit juices. One of your cousins sits next to you and places a large plate of potato chips and cookies on the table. He has also brought two cans of soda. He offers you a can and asks you to share the snacks with him. What will you tell him?

Name ______________________ Class ______________ Date ____________

Skills Worksheet

Decision-Making Skills

Lesson: Managing Your Emotions

Read the following situation. Then, follow the steps below to decide what you would do in this situation.

You are at an amusement park with some friends. Your friends suggest you try the new roller coaster at the park. You are terribly afraid of roller coasters and you don't want to ride one. Your friend Sam starts teasing you about your fear. Anger starts to well up inside of you. You know Sam has hit your trigger. You want to hit or push him, however, you know that will only make matters worse.

1. **Identify the problem.** What decision do you have to make?

____

____

2. **Consider your values.** What is important to you?

____

____

3. **List the options.** What possible actions could you take?

____

____

4. **Weigh the consequences.** List the pros and cons of each option.

____

____

5. **Decide and act.** Describe what you will do. Explain your decision.

____

____

6. **Evaluate your choice.** How do you feel about the action you took? Did you make a good decision? Would you take a different action if faced with the same scenario again?

____

____

Name ______________________ Class ______________ Date ____________

Skills Worksheet

Decision-Making Skills

Lesson: Getting Help

Read the following situation. Then, write a letter to José and explain some of the things he could do to encourage his mom to get help. Be sure to include some decision-making skills in your letter to José.

José is feeling very upset these days. His mother cries for no real reason and doesn't want to spend time with José and his brother. Some mornings, they don't see her at all because she just stays in bed. When they ask her if there's anything wrong, she gets mad, goes to the bedroom, and stays there for hours.

Name ______________________ Class ______________ Date ____________

Skills Worksheet

Refusal Skills

Lesson: Expressing Emotions

Describe how you would use the following refusal skills to respond to the following scenario. Remember to be clear and choose your words carefully. Describe your body language as well as your words.

You are very sad because your dog just died. You have decided to go to a party with some of your friends. You don't want to talk about being sad because you think that some of your friends would think you were being ridiculous. One of your friends notices that you are sad and offers you a beer. She tells you that drinking a beer will make you feel better.

1. **Say no.** How would you say no to your friend?

   ____

   ____

2. **Offer an alternative.** What else could you do to get over your sadness?

   ____

   ____

3. **Stand your ground.** What would you do if your friend kept pressuring you to drink the beer?

   ____

   ____

4. **Walk away.** Describe how you would get out of the situation.

   ____

   ____

5. **Plan ahead.** What could you do to avoid this situation?

   ____

   ____

6. **Have a support system.** Who will stand by you when you are in this situation? How can you use these people as support when dealing with this situation?

   ____

   ____

Name ______________________ Class ____________ Date ____________

Skills Worksheet

Refusal Skills

Lesson: Managing Your Emotions

Imagine that you are the advice columnist for a city newspaper. You must answer the following letter to Rob, who needs help managing stress. Be sure to include refusal skills that Rob can use to deal with his friend Tom.

Dear Ms. Igivehelp,

I was moved to a new middle school because I had good grades and this school is more challenging. But I find all of the classes to be so hard. It takes so much time to keep up with my homework and play on the basketball team. It's really hard to make friends here, and I am so stressed out. My best friend Tom from my old school wants me to run away from home. He thinks if I do that my parents will get scared and let me go back to my old school, but I know that will only make things worse. I feel like Tom is my only friend left right now, but how do I tell him no?

Please help,

Rob

Name ______________________________ Class ______________ Date ____________

Skills Worksheet

Decision-Making Skills

Lesson: Stress Is Only Natural

Imagine that you are an advice columnist for a newspaper. Read the following letter sent to you and respond by helping the reader make a good decision.

Dear Know-It-All,

I just finished reading an article about stress and stressors in my favorite teen magazine. The article said that if something is causing you stress, you have to stop doing it immediately. It also said that it's extremely dangerous to your health to do anything that might cause you stress. It said that if you keep all stress out of your life, you will be healthier. My question is this: Is it possible to keep stress out of your life? I'm trying my best to follow this advice, but now I'm so anxious to avoid stress, that things I didn't even think twice about before are bothering me. This is going on all day, every day, until I'm just exhausted.

Please help,

Distressed

Dear Distressed,

____

____

____

____

____

____

____

____

____

____

____

____

____

Stress Is Only Natural,

Know-It-All

Name ______________________ Class ______________ Date ______________

Skills Worksheet

Decision-Making Skills

Lesson: Managing Distress

Read the following situation. Then, follow the steps below to decide what you would do in this situation.

You and three other teens joined the school drama club at the beginning of the school year and became friends. At first, it seemed like all of you were being ignored for the best parts and were required to spend too much time on boring tasks. A few weeks ago, you decided to reframe the situation and try to change your distressful experience by looking at it from another point of view. It's been working and you're relieved to realize that joining was a good decision and that the hard work and lack of recognition at the outset were a part of the total experience. Unfortunately, the other three new club members are still stuck in a distressful situation, and now they want to go to the principal to make a formal complaint about how they've been treated. You don't feel the same way anymore, but you want to help them.

1. **Identify the problem.** What decision do you have to make?

   ____

2. **Consider your values.** What is important to you?

   ____

   ____

3. **List the options.** What possible actions could you take?

   ____

   ____

4. **Weigh the consequences.** List the pros and cons of each option.

   ____

   ____

5. **Decide and act.** Describe what you will do. Explain your decision.

   ____

   ____

6. **Evaluate your choice.** How do you feel about the action you took? Did you make a good decision? Would you take a different action if faced with the same scenario again?

   ____

   ____

Name ______________________ Class ______________ Date ____________

Skills Worksheet

Refusal Skills

Lesson: Stress Is Only Natural

Describe how you would use the following refusal skills to respond to the following scenario. Remember to be clear and choose your words carefully. Describe your body language as well as your words.

Your best friend, Pat, has been going to the same summer camp ever since he turned six and plans on going again this summer. This year he'll be in the teen program in which campers get to canoe across the lake and camp outside for two nights. Pat can't think about anything else. In fact, he can barely do his schoolwork or sleep at night he's so excited. Now, he's decided that you have to come along to "have the best time of our lives." You don't want to go. You feel kind of sick every time Pat asks if you've filled out the application yet. You don't want to let your friend down and that's bothering you, too. Now, *you* can't concentrate on your homework or get to sleep at night!

1. **Say no.** How would you say no to Pat?

 ____

2. **Offer an alternative.** What else could you do with Pat?

 ____

 ____

3. **Stand your ground.** What would you do if Pat kept pressuring you?

 ____

 ____

4. **Walk away.** Describe how you would get out of the situation.

 ____

 ____

5. **Plan ahead.** What could you do to avoid this situation? Who can help you practice refusing this action?

 ____

 ____

6. **Have a support system.** Who will stand by you when you make this decision? How can you use these people as support when refusing to do this action?

 ____

 ____

Name _______________ Class _______________ Date _______________

Skills Worksheet

Refusal Skills

Lesson: Defense Mechanisms

Read the following scenario. Then, write an ending to the scenario on the lines below. Explain how you will use refusal skills in this situation.

You've known Chris since kindergarten. Chris always threw temper tantrums if she didn't get her way, but lately she's really been out of control. The other day she actually grabbed your wrist and tried to pull you away from a group of friends. She's openly critical of your other friends and it's getting to a point where no one wants her around, but you keep making excuses for her because you know that telling her you agree with the others will be really difficult. You've been trying for months to ignore the situation hoping that it would change. The school trip is coming up and no one will talk with you if you sit with Chris. Chris is pressuring you to sign up to sit with her; your other friends are pressuring you to sit with them. You're going to have to fix this problem.

Name ______________________ Class ______________ Date ____________

Skills Worksheet

Decision-Making Skills

Lesson: Building Relationships

Read the following situation. Then, follow the steps below to decide what you would do in this situation.

Your best friend Ray is not as good in math as you are. The big math test is tomorrow. Your math class will take the test before Ray's, and Ray has asked you to try to remember as many of the test questions as you can and to tell him what they are at lunch. That way Ray will get a head start on the answers before he takes the test.

1. **Identify the problem.** What decision do you have to make?

____

____

2. **Consider your values.** What is important to you?

____

____

3. **List the options.** What possible actions could you take?

____

____

4. **Weigh the consequences.** List the pros and cons of each option.

____

____

5. **Decide and act.** Describe what you will do. Explain your decision.

____

____

6. **Evaluate your choice.** How do you feel about the action you took? Did you make a good decision? Would you take a different action if faced with the same scenario again?

____

____

Name ______________________ Class ______________ Date ______________

Skills Worksheet

Decision-Making Skills

Lesson: Practicing Abstinence

Read the following situation. Then, follow the steps below to decide what you would do in this situation.

Emily is worried because her friend Karen has been hanging around with people who are pressuring her to take risks. One of the boys in the group, Keith, has asked Karen to come to a party on Friday. No adults will be at the party. Karen knows that her parents would not approve. If you were Emily, how would you help Karen make a good decision?

1. **Identify the problem.** What decision do you have to make?

____

____

2. **Consider your values.** What is important to you?

____

____

3. **List the options.** What possible actions could you take?

____

____

4. **Weigh the consequences.** List the pros and cons of each option.

____

____

5. **Decide and act.** Describe what you will do. Explain your decision.

____

____

6. **Evaluate your choice.** How do you feel about the action you took? Did you make a good decision? Would you take a different action if faced with the same scenario again?

____

____

Name ______________________ Class ______________ Date ____________

Skills Worksheet

Refusal Skills

Lesson: Family Relationships

Describe how you would use the following refusal skills to respond to the following scenario. Remember to be clear and choose your words carefully. Describe your body language as well as your words.

Your older sister Katie has some after-school chores to do. But she never seems to have the time to do them. About a month ago, she began asking you to do her chores for her, but you have your own chores to do as well as your homework. Katie is really pressuring you lately to take on these added responsibilities.

1. **Say no.** How would you say no to Katie?

____

____

2. **Offer an alternative.** What else could you do for Katie?

____

____

3. **Stand your ground.** What would you do if Katie kept pressuring your to do her chores?

____

____

4. **Walk away.** Describe how you would get out of the situation.

____

____

5. **Plan ahead.** What could you do to avoid this situation? Who can help you practice refusing this action?

____

____

6. **Have a support system.** Who will stand by you when you make this decision? How can you use these people as support when refusing to do this action?

____

____

Name ________________________ Class ____________ Date ____________

Skills Worksheet

Refusal Skills

Lesson: Practicing Abstinence

Describe how you would use the following refusal skills to respond to the following scenario. Remember to be clear and choose your words carefully. Describe your body language as well as your words.

John has asked Meg out on a third date. Meg really likes John. They've both been waiting weeks to see this movie. It's a great night. The movie is funny, and they have a wonderful time. On the way home, John suggests a walk through a darkened park. Meg feels nervous, but she knows she can trust John to take care of her. In the park, John asks her to be his girlfriend and go with him to the school dance. Then John kisses her and puts his hands in places that make her uncomfortable. Meg asks him to stop but he doesn't. When she pushes him away, he says angrily, "Hey, you're my girlfriend now. You can't push me away."

1. **Say no.** How can Meg say no to John?

____

2. **Offer an alternative.** Other than argue with John, what else can Meg do ?

____

____

3. **Stand your ground.** What can Meg do if John keeps pressuring her to do things that make her uncomfortable?

____

____

4. **Walk away.** Describe how Meg can get out of the situation.

____

____

5. **Plan ahead.** What could Meg do to avoid this situation? Who can help her practice refusing this action?

____

____

6. **Have a support system.** Who might stand by Meg when she makes this decision? How can Meg use these people as support when refusing to do this action?

____

____

Name ______________________ Class ______________ Date ____________

Skills Worksheet

Decision-Making Skills

Lesson: What Is Conflict?

Read the following situation. Then, follow the steps below to decide what you would do in this situation.

Your classmate Ray has an older brother who has been riding his bicycle right behind you as you walk home from school. It often feels like he is going to run into you, especially if you walk too slowly. You've asked him to stop but he just laughs in response. One of your friends has offered to take care of the situation by doing the same thing to Ray.

1. **Identify the problem.** What decision do you have to make?

____

____

2. **Consider your values.** What is important to you?

____

____

3. **List the options.** What possible actions could you take?

____

____

____

4. **Weigh the consequences.** List the pros and cons of each option.

____

____

5. **Decide and act.** Describe what you will do. Explain your decision.

____

____

6. **Evaluate your choice.** How do you feel about the action you took? Did you make a good decision? Would you take a different action if faced with the same scenario again?

____

____

____

Name ______________________ Class ______________ Date ____________

Skills Worksheet

Decision-Making Skills

Lesson: Getting Help for Conflicts

Read the following situation. Then, finish the story using decision-making skills.

You and your cousin Leah always spend a lot of time together doing different activities during summer vacation. This year, however, when you call Leah to make summer plans, she says that she has decided to do something else and has already made other plans. You ask Leah for an explanation, but she doesn't give you one and you hang up the phone on her abruptly. You call Leah again several times, but she won't take your calls.

Name ______________________ Class ______________ Date ____________

Skills Worksheet

Refusal Skills

Lesson: Communicating During Conflicts

Describe how you would use the following refusal skills to respond to the following scenario. Remember to be clear and to choose your words carefully. Describe your body language as well as your words.

You and Joanne have been working on a school project that is due tomorrow and have just enough time after school today to finish the project so you can do the rest of your homework after dinner. As you are leaving school to go to the library, your friends Steven and Chris invite you and Joanne to join them for pizza. Joanne immediately accepts their invitation. She then turns to you and says "Are you coming with us?"

1. **Say no.** How would you say no to this invitation?

____

____

2. **Offer an alternative.** What other plans could make with your friends?

____

____

3. **Stand your ground.** What would you do if Joanne insists that you join your friends for pizza?

____

____

4. **Walk away.** Describe how you would get out of the situation.

____

____

5. **Plan ahead.** What could you do to avoid this situation? Who can help you practice refusing this action?

____

____

6. **Have a support system.** Who will stand by you when you make this decision? How can you use these people as support when refusing to do this action?

____

____

Name ______________________ Class ______________ Date ____________

Skills Worksheet

Refusal Skills

Lesson: Preventing Violence

Describe how you would use the following refusal skills to respond to the following scenario. Remember to be clear and to choose your words carefully. Describe your body language as well as your words.

A student at school has been teasing you all year long. This time he has gone too far by making fun of you in front of someone you really like. Other students have heard your argument and have gathered around you. You hear shouts encouraging you to hit him.

1. **Say no.** How would you say no to this action?

____

____

2. **Offer an alternative.** What could you do to avoid a violent conflict?

____

____

3. **Stand your ground.** What would you do if the other student insists on fighting?

____

____

____

4. **Walk away.** Describe how you would get out of the situation.

____

____

____

5. **Plan ahead.** What could you do to avoid this situation? Who can help you practice refusing this action?

____

____

6. **Have a support system.** Who will stand by you when you make this decision? How can you use these people as support when refusing to do this action?

____

____

Name ______________________ Class ______________ Date ____________

Skills Worksheet

Decision-Making Skills

Lesson: Why People Use Tobacco

Read the following situation. Then, follow the steps below to decide what you would do in this situation.

Your older brother, Doug, smokes. You admire your older brother, who's really cool and popular. You often walk home with him and his friends. Usually, Doug or one of his friends offers you a cigarette. And you always refuse. After the friends are gone, you tell Doug that you really don't want to start smoking. Doug laughs and tells you that you're too young to become hooked on cigarettes. Doug tells you that you should at least get used to smoking a few cigarettes because it is expected and will make you popular.

1. **Identify the problem.** What decision do you have to make?

   ____

   ____

2. **Consider your values.** What is important to you?

   ____

   ____

3. **List your options.** What possible actions could you take?

   ____

   ____

4. **Weigh the consequences.** List the pros and cons of each option.

   ____

   ____

5. **Decide and act.** Describe what you will do. Explain your reasons.

   ____

   ____

6. **Evaluate your choice.** How do you feel about the action you took? Did you make a good decision? Would you take a different action if faced with the same scenario again?

   ____

   ____

Name ______________________ Class ______________ Date ____________

Skills Worksheet

Decision-Making Skills

Lesson: Choosing Not to Use Tobacco

Read the following dramatic scene. Then, write the final dialogue for Shari.

LAURA: The party Saturday night was so great! It's too bad you were too sick to come. We had a blast.

SHARI: Was the whole crowd there? Even Mark?

LAURA: Everyone was there. It was terrific. Yeah, Mark was there—alone. But he danced a lot with Maria. (Laura takes a cigarette out of her bag, lights it, and begins smoking.)

SHARI: When did you start smoking?

LAURA: Only at parties! You know, someone always offers you a cigarette at parties. So I take it. I mean, it's only to have fun at a party.

SHARI: Yeah, but we're not at a party now. Why are you smoking?

LAURA: I don't know. I just feel like it. (She sees Shari looking at her in disbelief.) I'm not becoming a smoker or anything. I just like to smoke a cigarette now and then.

SHARI: Come on, Laura, we always said smoking was stupid. Now here you are smoking cigarettes. And it's not just at parties. It's here. You're becoming a smoker.

LAURA: No, I'm not. It's just now and then. Anyway, I'm too young to get addicted. I can stop any time I want. And, you know, smoking doesn't harm you when you're young. It's only bad if you keep smoking when you're old. So, please, don't worry about me, okay?

SHARI:

Name ______________________ Class ______________ Date ____________

Skills Worksheet

Refusal Skills

Lesson: Quitting

Describe how you would use the following refusal skills to respond to the following scenario. Remember to be clear and choose your words carefully. Describe your body language as well as your words.

One year ago, you started smoking. You have since regretted it and decided to quit. You have not smoked in three weeks. You are feeling really well physically and you are also feeling strong psychologically. It makes you feel good to know that you have the willpower to give up cigarettes. However, when your friends come over for the evening, it is always a trial because Denise and Tammy both still smoke. On this evening, you're all having a good time, but Denise and Tammy keep pushing you to take a few puffs on their cigarettes. You don't want to, but it gets hard to refuse, especially when Tammy holds a lit cigarette out to you and says, "Come on, you know how much you liked to smoke."

1. **Say no.** How would you say no to Tammy?

____

____

2. **Offer an alternative.** What else could you suggest to your friends who smoke?

____

____

3. **Stand your ground.** What would you do if they kept pressuring you to smoke?

____

____

4. **Walk away.** Describe how you would get out of the situation.

____

____

5. **Plan ahead.** What could you to to avoid this situation? Who can help you practice refusing this action?

____

6. **Have a support system.** Who will stand by you when you make this decision? How can you use these people as support when refusing to do this action?

____

Name ______________________ Class ____________ Date ____________

Skills Worksheet

Refusal Skills

Lesson: Choosing Not to Use Tobacco

You are the "Know-It-All" of your school newspaper. Students write you letters asking for advice, and you reply by giving them advice in your newspaper column. You receive the letter below from a troubled student at your school. Use the refusal skills you have learned to reply to the letter. Tell the student how to "say no," "stand his ground," "walk away," "plan ahead," and "have a support system." Describe to the student how he may offer an alternative to the problem.

Dear Know-It-All,

I'm a student at this school and I really like it and the people here. My problem is that there is one group of students who offer me cigarettes after school, and I don't want to smoke. They make fun of me for not taking a cigarette. Sometimes, I make a joke out of it, but that doesn't help much. Sometimes, I tell them that I want to be on the school running team, so I can't smoke. I mean, nobody who smokes will ever win a race, right?

Most of my friends don't really want to smoke either, but they take the cigarettes anyway when someone offers them. My friends say they aren't worried because one cigarette won't hurt. They do it just to be hanging out with that group of students. They tell me to just take a cigarette and not worry. But I really don't want to. What should I do?

Thanks for your help,

Hold-out

Dear Hold-out,

____

____

____

____

____

____

____

____

____

Good luck,

Know-It-All

Name ______________________ Class ______________ Date ____________

Skills Worksheet

Decision-Making Skills

Lesson: Alcohol, You, and Other People

Read the following situation. Then, follow the steps below to decide what you would do in this situation.

You've been invited to a party at a classmate's home after the Friday evening pep rally. You've checked to be sure there will be an adult chaperone so that you can assure your parents that there will be no drinking at the party. When you get to the party, your classmate's parents are home just as you were told they would be, but there's a keg of beer in the kitchen and other kids are drinking.

1. **Identify the problem.** What decision do you have to make?

____

____

2. **Consider your values.** What is important to you?

____

____

3. **List the options.** What possible actions could you take?

____

____

____

4. **Weigh the consequences.** List the pros and cons of each option.

____

____

5. **Decide and act.** Describe what you will do. Explain your decision.

____

____

6. **Evaluate your choice**. How do you feel about the action you took? Did you make a good decision? Would you take a different action if faced with the same scenario again?

____

____

____

Name ________________________________ Class ________________ Date ______________

Skills Worksheet

Decision-Making Skills

Lesson: Alternatives to Alcohol

Make a one-page print public service announcement (PSA) promoting ways to use time productively instead of destructively. Your PSA message should help teens make the important decision not to drink. In your PSA, recommend alternatives to drinking alcohol that can offer teens the enjoyment and a sense of personal fulfillment they need to help them successfully resist the pressure to drink. Use graphics to support your text. When you are finished, answer the following question.

What activities does your PSA suggest, and why are they good alternatives to drinking?

Name ______________________ Class ______________ Date ____________

Skills Worksheet

Refusal Skills

Lesson: Drunk Driving

Describe how you would use the following refusal skills to respond to the following scenario. Remember to choose your words carefully. Describe your body language as well as your words.

Your friend Chris's sister is giving Chris a ride home from an after school activity. When Chris's sister arrives, she offers you a ride home too. Just as you are about to get in the car, Chris's sister offers you and Chris a drink from a can of beer that she's been drinking.

1. **Say no.** How would you say no to Chris's sister's invitation?

____

____

2. **Offer an alternative.** What could you do instead?

____

____

3. **Stand your ground.** What would you do if Chris's sister kept pressuring you to have a drink and accept her offer of a ride home? What would you do if Chris also pressured you to accept his sister's invitations?

____

____

4. **Walk away.** Describe how you would get out of the situation.

____

____

5. **Plan ahead.** What could you do to avoid this situation? Who can help you practice refusing this action?

____

____

6. **Have a support system.** Who will stand by you when make this decision? How can you use these people as support when refusing to do this action?

____

____

Name ______________________ Class ______________ Date ______________

Skills Worksheet

Refusal Skills

Lesson: Resisting the Pressure to Drink

Someone with a drinking problem often rationalizes or minimizes his or her behavior or blames it on someone or something else and then looks to other people to validate his or her behavior. For each of the statements below write a realistic rebuttal.

1. **One drink won't hurt me.** (minimizing)

____

____

2. **The only way to have fun is to drink.** (rationalizing)

____

____

3. **I drink only because I'm so stressed out.** (blaming)

____

____

4. **I just want to see what drinking is like.** (minimizing)

____

____

5. **Drinking makes my problems go away.** (rationalizing)

____

____

6. **If my parents didn't yell so much, I wouldn't drink.** (blaming)

____

____

7. **I drink only at parties.** (minimizing)

____

____

8. **All of my friends drink.** (rationalizing)

____

____

Name ______________________ Class ______________ Date ____________

Skills Worksheet

Decision-Making Skills

Lesson: The Consequences of Drug Abuse

Read the following situation. Then, follow the steps below to decide what you would do in this situation.

Lately you've noticed that your friend Lori has been distant. She doesn't want to come to the mall with you and Jill, and she missed volleyball practice three times this week. Lori has been spending more time with her friend Mike, but even that wouldn't explain why she dropped a whole letter grade in math and English. Jill says that she overheard girls in the lunch-line saying that Mike and his friends use drugs. Jill is concerned that Lori is using drugs too and she thinks the two of you should tell Lori's parents or a teacher.

1. **Identify the problem.** What decision do you have to make?

____

____

2. **Consider your values.** What is important to you?

____

____

3. **List the options.** What possible actions could you take?

____

____

4. **Weigh the consequences.** List the pros and cons of each option.

____

____

____

5. **Decide and act.** Describe what you will do. Explain your decision.

____

____

6. **Evaluate your choice.** How do you feel about the action you took? Did you make a good decision? Would you take a different action if faced with the same scenario again?

____

____

Name ______________________ Class ______________ Date ____________

Skills Worksheet

Decision-Making Skills

Lesson: Staying Drug Free

Finish the following story, explaining how you would make your decision, and what it would be.

It's Saturday night and the end of the school year! You and your friend Bart have been invited to three different parties. The party at Phil's house could be trouble because his parents are out of town and people say that Phil drinks alcohol. When Bart learns that Mandy is at Phil's party, Bart insists that you go there with him. You remind Bart that your parents would not allow you to go to a party that might have alcohol. "So what?" Bart says. "We don't have to drink. Let's go. I really want to see Mandy." Still, you hesitate. If your parents find out you went to Phil's party, you could be grounded for the summer.

Name ______________________ Class ______________ Date ____________

Skills Worksheet

Refusal Skills

Lesson: Drug Misuse and Abuse

Describe how you would use the following refusal skills to respond to the following scenario. Remember to be clear and choose your words carefully. Describe your body language as well as your words.

You have a cold. During soccer practice, you've been having difficulty breathing while doing sprints. After practice, you meet your friend Taylor and walk home together as always. You tell Taylor about your breathing problem and gripe, "If only I could beat this cold." Taylor has asthma and she offers you one of her prescription inhalers to use. "But it's your prescription," you say. "So?" she answers. "Just use it until your cold goes away. Why suffer?"

1. **Say no.** How would you say no to Taylor?

   ____

   ____

2. **Offer an alternative.** What else could you do about your breathing?

   ____

   ____

3. **Stand your ground.** What would you do if Taylor kept pressuring you to use her inhaler?

   ____

   ____

4. **Walk away.** Describe how you would get out of the situation.

   ____

   ____

5. **Plan ahead.** What could you do to avoid this situation? Who could help you practice refusing this action?

   ____

   ____

6. **Have a support system.** Who will stand by you when you make this decision? How can you use these people as support when refusing to do this action?

   ____

   ____

Name ______________________ Class ______________ Date ______________

Skills Worksheet

Refusal Skills

Lesson: Staying Drug Free

Describe how you would use the following refusal skills to respond to the following scenario. Remember to be clear and choose your words carefully. Describe your body language as well as your words.

Devon's parents are out of town. After the football game, he invites a group of people to his house to celebrate the team's victory. You and your friends stop for some cheeseburgers and then go to Devon's house. The music is blaring, people are dancing, and everyone is in a good mood. However, when you go into the kitchen to say hi to some other friends, you see that they are smoking marijuana. They grin and pass the marijuana to you.

1. **Say no.** How would you say no to your friends?

____

____

2. **Offer an alternative.** What else could you do with your friends?

____

____

____

3. **Stand your ground.** What would you do if they kept pressuring you to smoke?

____

____

4. **Walk away.** Describe how you would get out of the situation.

____

____

5. **Plan ahead.** What could you do to avoid this situation? Who can help you practice refusing this action?

____

____

6. **Have a support system.** Who will stand by you when you make this decision? How can you use these people as support when refusing to do this action?

____

____

Name ______________________ Class ______________ Date ____________

Skills Worksheet

Decision-Making Skills

Lesson: Bacterial Infections

Read the following situation. Then, follow the steps below to decide what you would do in this situation.

You awaken on a Saturday morning with congestion, a sore throat, and a cough. You're pretty sure you have a cold, and your parents agree. You have plans for later that day to attend a party to celebrate your best friend Jamal's birthday. You know that the party is important to Jamal, and that your attendance will mean a lot to him. You spend the morning working on some homework and straightening up your room. After having a bowl of soup for lunch, you're feeling pretty good—except for your sore throat. You've also noticed that your nose has started to run. While you're washing out your bowl, the phone rings. It's Jamal.

1. **Identify the problem.** What decision do you have to make?

____

____

2. **Consider your values.** What is important to you?

____

____

3. **List the options.** What possible actions could you take?

____

____

4. **Weigh the consequences.** List the pros and cons of each option.

____

____

5. **Decide and act.** Describe what you will do. Explain your decision.

____

____

6. **Evaluate your choice.** How do you feel about the action you took? Did you make a good decision? Would you take a different action if faced with the same scenario again?

____

____

Name ______________________ Class ______________ Date ____________

Skills Worksheet

Decision-Making Skills

Lesson: Viral Infections

Read each of the following situations and choose one. Then, on a separate sheet of paper, describe the possible consequences of the decision you made in response to the situation.

1. For the past two days, you've had a runny nose, a slight fever, and a headache. You're pretty sure you have a cold. However, when you describe your symptoms to a friend, he mentions that your symptoms sound similar to his symptoms when he had a sinus infection. He encourages you to tell your parents so they can take you to see your doctor. You don't feel like going to the doctor, so you don't ask your parents to make an appointment for you. You decide that you're just going to treat this like a cold and wait for the symptoms to pass.

2. After school one day, your family attends a book reading at the local library. Following the book reading, your sister introduces you to several of her friends. Conscious of minding your manners, you greet each of her friends with a handshake and polite conversation. In addition to your sister's friends, you also shake hands with the author, a librarian, five or six of your schoolmates, and two of your teachers. When you get home, your father reminds you to wash your hands before dinner. You're really hungry and anxious to get to the table, so you decide to quickly rinse your hands under some cold water.

3. A neighborhood friend, Al, has been diagnosed with mononucleosis. You recently spent some time with Al, and you remember that he sneezed once or twice while you were with him that day. Some of your other friends told their parents about Al, and their parents took them to their doctors to be tested for mononucleosis. You don't have any symptoms of mononucleosis, though, so you decide not to alert your parents.

Name ______________________ Class ____________ Date ____________

Skills Worksheet

Refusal Skills

Lesson: Sexually Transmitted Diseases

Describe how to use refusal skills to respond to the following scenario. Remember to be clear and choose your words carefully. Describe your body language as well as your words.

Your best friend tells you about her date with her boyfriend and asks you for advice. She and her date were at the movies and he was pressuring her to have sex later. She reminded him that not wanting to catch an STD was only one of the reasons she didn't want to have sex. Her date insists that he doesn't have any symptoms of STDs. He also suggested that she could just take some medicine if she caught an STD. Your friend knows that the only sure way to protect herself from any STD is by practicing abstinence, but her date still wants to have sex and insists that there is no great risk to her health.

1. **Say no.** How could your friend say no to the person she is dating?

____

____

2. **Offer an alternative.** What else could she do with this person?

____

____

3. **Stand your ground.** What should your friend do if he keeps pressuring her to ignore her worries about STDs?

____

____

4. **Walk away.** Describe how she could get out of the situation.

____

____

5. **Plan ahead.** What could your friend do to avoid this situation? Who can help her practice refusing this action?

____

____

6. **Have a support system.** Who will stand by your friend when she makes this decision? How can she use these people as support when refusing to do this action?

____

____

Name ______________________ Class ______________ Date ____________

Skills Worksheet

Refusal Skills

Lesson: Preventing the Spread of Infectious Diseases

Describe how you would use the following refusal skills to respond to the following scenario. Remember to be clear and choose your words carefully. Describe your body language as well as your words.

You and your friends are at your house on a Friday night. Everyone is watching a rented video while enjoying some pizza and drinks. You're sitting on the couch, drinking a glass of orange-pineapple juice. During the movie, you see your friend Allison taking a sip from her boyfriend's glass of milk. After the movie, Allison comes over and asks how your juice is. She then asks if she can have a sip out of your glass to see if she likes it.

1. **Say no.** How would you say no to Allison?

____

____

2. **Offer an alternative.** What other option could you offer to Allison?

____

____

3. **Stand your ground.** What would you do if Allison kept pressuring you to let her drink from your glass?

____

____

4. **Walk away.** Describe how you would get out of the situation.

____

____

5. **Plan ahead.** What could you do to avoid this situation? Who can help you practice refusing this action?

____

____

6. **Have a support system.** Who will stand by you when you make this decision? How can you use these people as support when refusing to do this action?

____

____

Name ______________________ Class ______________ Date ____________

Skills Worksheet

Decision-Making Skills

Lesson: Digestive System

Read the following situation. Then, follow the steps below to decide what you would do in this situation.

Your doctor has told you that you have celiac disease. He explained that your body is allergic to a protein called gluten. You found out that gluten is found in grains, such as wheat, rye, and barley. The doctor advised you not to eat foods that contain these grains. Pizza is one of the foods you should not eat. After a game, your friends invite you to share a pizza with them.

1. **Identify the problem.** What decision do you have to make?

____

____

____

2. **Consider your values.** What is important to you?

____

____

____

3. **List the options**. What possible actions could you take?

____

____

4. **Weigh the consequences.** List the pros and cons of each option.

____

____

5. **Decide and act.** Describe what you will do. Explain your decision.

____

____

6. **Evaluate your choice.** How do you feel about the action you took? Did you make a good decision? Would you take a different action if faced with the same scenario again?

____

____

Name ______________________ Class ______________ Date ____________

Skills Worksheet

Decision-Making Skills

Lesson: Eyes and Ears

Imagine that you are a reporter for your school paper. Your assignment this month is to write the advice column. Answer the following letter from a fellow student.

Dear Know-It-All:

My dad noticed that I was squinting when I was watching TV. He made an appointment with the eye doctor to have my eyes checked. Sure enough, I now have to wear glasses.

I have a problem, though. My family thinks I look great in my new glasses, and I do admit I can see better. But I'm worried that my classmates will tease me when they see me wearing my glasses. I just don't want to wear my glasses in school. What should I do?

Near Sighted

Dear Near Sighted: ____

Name ______________________ Class ______________ Date ____________

Skills Worksheet

Refusal Skills

Lesson: Respiratory System

Describe how you would use the following refusal skills to respond to the following scenario. Remember to be clear and choose your words carefully. Describe your body language as well as your words.

When you visited your grandfather during the school vacation, you noticed that he had difficulty breathing. Grandma told you that he had emphysema. His doctor said that the disease was caused by smoking cigarettes. It made you sad to see how smoking had made life so difficult for a person you loved dearly. You remember this experience when your friend Larry invites you and Jill to smoke with him. Jill accepts his invitation, expecting that you will, too.

1. **Say no.** How would you say no to Larry and Jill?

____

____

2. **Offer an alternative.** What else could you do with Larry and Jill?

____

____

3. **Stand your ground.** What would do if they kept pressuring you to smoke?

____

____

4. **Walk away.** Describe how you would get out of the situation.

____

____

5. **Plan ahead.** What could you do to avoid this situation? Who can help you practice refusing this action?

____

____

6. **Have a support system.** Who will stand by you when you make this decision? How can you use these people as support when refusing to do this action?

____

____

Name ______________________ Class ______________ Date ______________

Skills Worksheet

Refusal Skills

Lesson: Nervous System

Complete the following scenario showing how Jeff can use refusal skills in a risky situation.

Gil and Meg invited Jeff to go bike riding with them around the park. At the meeting place, Jeff notices that they are not wearing helmets. Gil mentions that he feels free without his helmet. "I like to take risks," he says. Jeff shakes his head in disbelief but can see that it will be hard to convince Gil, who was already maneuvering to race ahead of him on the road. He signals Jeff to race with him, even though the traffic on the road is heavy.

Name ______________________ Class ____________ Date ____________

Skills Worksheet

Decision-Making Skills

Lesson: The Male Reproductive System

Read the following situation. Then, follow the steps to decide what you would do in this situation.

You are at a friend's house for the day. Your friend and all of the guys in the neighborhood have decided to play football. You don't have any of your protective gear with you. Your friend encourages you to play anyway.

1. **Identify the problem.** What decision do you have to make?

____

____

2. **Consider your values.** What is important to you?

____

____

3. **List the options.** What possible actions could you take?

____

____

4. **Weigh the consequences.** List the pros and cons of each option.

____

____

5. **Decide and act.** Describe what you will do. Explain your decision.

____

____

6. **Evaluate your choice.** How do you feel about the action you took? Did you make a good decision? Would you take a different action if faced with the same scenario again?

____

____

Name ______________________ Class ______________ Date ____________

Skills Worksheet

Decision-Making Skills

Lesson: The Female Reproductive System

Read the following situations. For each, predict three consequences of the decision that is described. Remember that consequences can be positive or negative.

1. Marta has questions about the way her body is changing. She is sure that something is wrong with her health because she suffers such severe menstrual cramps each month. In fact, she misses a few days of school each month due to menstrual cramps. Marta has decided not to tell her doctor about her problem because she is too embarrassed to talk about it.

____

____

____

____

____

2. Tara's 20-year-old sister is in college. She has a busy schedule of classes, a job, and a lot of classwork. She has been so busy she has skipped her annual doctor's exams for the past two years.

____

____

____

____

____

3. Yolanda's body is not changing at the same rate as all of her friends' bodies. At first she was really worried. Then, Yolanda decided that whenever she had a question about her development she would ask her mother, rather than sit and worry.

____

____

____

____

____

Name ______________________ Class ______________ Date ____________

Skills Worksheet

Refusal Skills

Lesson: The Endocrine System

Describe how you would use the following refusal skills to respond to the following scenario. Remember to be clear and choose your words carefully. Describe your body language as well as your words.

You and your best friend, Greg, have been selected for the football team. Greg is quite a bit bigger than you. In fact, you are the smallest player on the team. One day, Greg offers you some tablets he purchased through the Internet. He says they contain growth hormones, and you'll see results in just a week. He places a few of the tablets in his hand, and tries to pass them to you.

1. **Say no.** How would you say no to Greg?

____

____

2. **Offer an alternative.** What else could you do to avoid taking the pills from Greg?

____

____

3. **Stand your ground.** What would you do if he kept pressuring you to take the tablets?

____

____

4. **Walk away.** Describe how you would get out of the situation.

____

____

5. **Plan ahead.** What could you do to avoid this situation? Who could help you practice refusing to take the tablets?

____

____

6. **Have a support system.** Who will stand by you when you make this decision? How can you use these people as support when refusing to take these tablets?

____

____

Name ______________________ Class ______________ Date ______________

Skills Worksheet

Refusal Skills

Lesson: Becoming an Adult

Imagine that you are the advice columnist at your school newspaper. Answer the following letters. Each of your answers must show how the writer can use refusal skills to avoid risky behavior.

1. Please help! My body is changing so much, and I feel so confused most of the time. One day I'm happy, and the next day I'm sad. My friend Lauren said I'd feel better if I had an alcoholic drink to relax. I sure would like to relax—is Lauren right?

____

____

____

____

2. I'm at the end of my rope. I just can't decide what I want to do with my life. My friend Jason has it all figured out. He is planning to be a doctor, and is already planning his class schedule so he can get into a good college. He has signed up for science camp this summer, and he's pressuring me to go with him. I'm pretty sure I'd rather go to music camp, but Jason already has my application form for science camp. How can I say no?

____

____

____

____

____

3. I really like to eat healthy foods, but I'm constantly getting teased about being a health nut. I know that eating well now will help me have good lifelong health, but my friends think that's the funniest thing they've ever heard. Tonight they're going out for fast food again. How can I say no without losing my friends?

____

____

____

____

Name ______________________________ Class ________________ Date ______________

Skills Worksheet

Decision-Making Skills

Lesson: Deciding to Give First Aid

Read the following situation. Then, follow the steps below to decide what you would do in this situation.

You and your friend Marta are alone at her house. She wants to build a new shelf for her bedroom, so she goes into the garage, where her father keeps wood and tools. Marta decides to use her father's saw, even though she is not supposed to do this without an adult. Unfortunately, her hand slips, and she gets a deep cut on her arm. Marta's father has a first aid kit in the garage. You have taken a first aid class, so you apply a piece of sterile gauze over the cut and put pressure on it. After a few minutes, however, the bleeding still hasn't stopped. You want to call for help, but Marta begs you not to. She is afraid that she will get in trouble.

1. **Identify the problem.** What decision do you have to make?

____

____

2. **Consider your values.** What is important to you?

____

____

3. **List the options.** What possible actions could you take?

____

____

4. **Weigh the consequences.** List the pros and cons of each option.

____

____

5. **Decide and act.** Describe what you will do. Explain your decision.

____

____

6. **Evaluate your choice.** How do you feel about the action you took? Did you make a good decision? Would you take a different action if faced with the same scenario again?

____

____

Name ______________________ Class ______________ Date ______________

Skills Worksheet

Decision-Making Skills

Lesson: Abdominal Thrusts and Rescue Breathing

Read the following situation. Then, follow the steps below to decide what you would do in this situation.

You and your older brother are at home alone eating dinner. Both of you are telling jokes and clowning around. Suddenly, your brother gets a funny look on his face and puts his hand to his throat. At first, you think he is just kidding, and you laugh. Then, you realize that he really is choking. Luckily, you took a first-aid class last month, so you know how to give abdominal thrusts. But you're afraid. What if you do something wrong?

1. **Identify the problem.** What decision do you have to make?

____

____

2. **Consider your values.** What is important to you?

____

____

3. **List the options.** What possible actions could you take?

____

____

4. **Weigh the consequences.** List the pros and cons of each option.

____

____

____

5. **Decide and act.** Describe what you will do. Explain your decision.

____

____

6. **Evaluate your choice.** How do you feel about the action you took? Did you make a good decision? Would you take a different action if faced with the same scenario again?

____

____

Name ______________________ Class ______________ Date ____________

Skills Worksheet

Refusal Skills

Lesson: Safety on the Road

Finish the story on the lines that follow. Help Tim use refusal skills to respond to Scott and Jenn. Describe Tim's body language and tone of voice as well as his words.

For Tim's birthday, his parents gave him a new bicycle helmet. He loved it. The helmet looked sharp, and he always liked getting new gear to use for cycling. The next afternoon, though, he met his friends Scott and Jenn at the park for a bike ride. Neither of them wore helmets, and they made fun of Tim for wearing one. They urged him to stash the helmet in the bushes and ride without it.

Name ______________________ Class ______________ Date ____________

Skills Worksheet

Refusal Skills

Lesson: Safety Outdoors

Describe how you would use refusal skills to respond to the following scenario. Remember to be clear and choose your words carefully. Describe your body language as well as your words.

Imagine that your class is spending a day at the lake. None of you has ever been to this spot before, but you're all having a great time swimming in a designated area. That afternoon, you and Mike wander away from the group, even though you're supposed to stay together. You find a big rock jutting out over the water. The rock is at least 20 feet high, and Mike dares you to dive from the top. When you say that sounds dangerous, Mike laughs and calls you a chicken.

1. **Say no.** How would you say no to Mike?

____

____

2. **Offer an alternative.** What else could you do with Mike?

____

____

3. **Stand your ground.** What would you do if Mike kept pressuring you to dive from the rock?

____

____

4. **Walk away.** Describe how you would get out of the situation.

____

____

5. **Plan ahead.** What could you do to avoid this situation?

____

____

6. **Have a support system.** Who will stand by you when you make this decision? How can you use these people as support when refusing to do this action?

____

____

9997257189 1 2 3 4 5 6